W9-CBU-210

Everything You Need to Know About

Sexual Identity

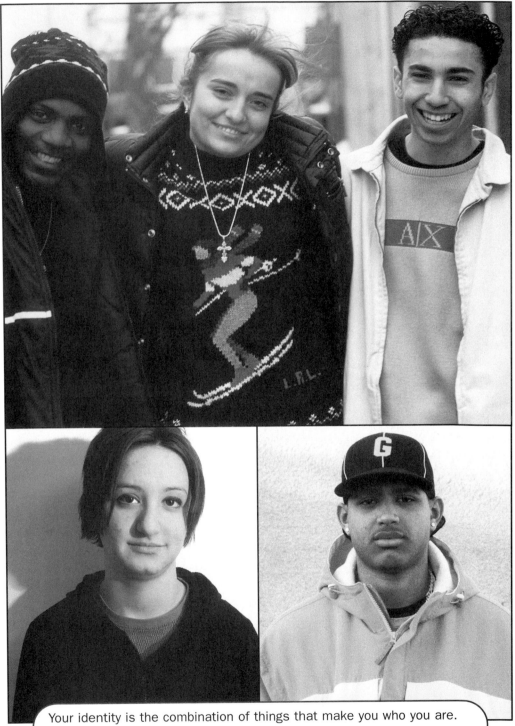

Your identity is the combination of things that make you who you are. It is how you see yourself and how you let other people see you.

Everything You Need to Know About

Sexual Identity

Jeff Donaldson-Forbes

The Rosen Publishing Group, Inc.
New York

In loving memory of Edward Heberger

Special thanks to Owen Borda of the Westchester County Department of Health for his input and advice.

Published in 2000 by The Rosen Publishing Group, Inc.
29 East 21st Street, New York, NY 10010

Library of Congress Cataloging-in-Publication Data

Donaldson-Forbes, Jeff.
   Everything you need to know about sexual identity / Jeff Donaldson-Forbes.
      p. cm.— (The need to know library)
   Includes bibliographical references and index.
   Summary: Describes the issue of sexual identity, providing insight on what it means to be heterosexual, bisexual, or homosexual.
   ISBN 0-8239-3089-0
   1. Sex instruction for teenagers. 2. Gender identity. 3. Sexual orientation. [1. Sex instruction for youth. 2. Sexual orientation.] I. Title. II. Series.

HQ35 .D64 2000
306.7—dc21   00-025495

Manufactured in the United States of America

Contents

Introduction: What
    Is Sexual Identity?   6

Chapter One   How Do I Know?   15

Chapter Two   Love and Sex   20

Chapter Three   Coming Out   32

Chapter Four   Someone to Look Up To   44

Chapter Five   The Life Ahead of You   52

Glossary   56

Where to Go for Help   58

For Further Reading   61

Index   62

Introduction: What Is Sexual Identity?

You are different from everyone else you know. No one else looks exactly like you do. No one else feels exactly the same things you do. Your identity is the combination of things that make you who you are. Your identity is how you see yourself and how you let other people see you—it is your personality.

Your Identity

Try to describe yourself. Are you male or female? Your gender—male or female—is a piece of your identity. What is your race? How old are you? Your age and race are other pieces of your identity. Think about your likes and dislikes. Do you like sports? Do you like foreign films? Do you prefer nighttime or daytime? Your answers to questions like these are also pieces of your identity.

Think about some other questions: What is your favorite subject at school? Do you know what kind of job you might like when you are an adult? Do you think you will marry and have children? There are no right or wrong answers to any of these questions. You have probably not decided about careers or marriage yet. All these pieces of your personality—and many more— make up your identity.

What Is Sexual Identity?

"Sexual identity" refers to a specific piece of your identity. Sexual identity describes whom you are attracted to with your feelings (emotional attraction) and your body (physical attraction). "Sexual preference" is another phrase that describes these attractions.

Emotional attraction is the desire to fall in love with someone. Emotional attraction draws you close to someone with feelings of love. Physical attraction is the desire you feel with your body. Physical attraction may be expressed by hugging or kissing. Sometimes having sex or making love is the result of physical attraction.

Have you ever dated? Have you ever had strong feelings for a boyfriend or girlfriend? Was that person male or female? If you have not dated, do you find yourself attracted to men or to women? If you do not find yourself feeling attracted to other people, that is OK. Attraction to other people occurs at different times in our lives, and not everyone feels attraction in the same way or all the time.

Who Are You Attracted To?

Most people in the world feel strong emotional and sexual attraction to people of the opposite sex. Most men are attracted to women. Most women are attracted to men. These people would define their sexual identity as heterosexual, or straight.

However, there are many people in the world who do not feel attracted emotionally or physically to people of the opposite sex. Many people in the world are attracted to people of the same sex. Many women are emotionally and physically attracted to other women. Many men are attracted in those ways to other men. These people would define their sexual identity as homosexual. Homosexual people are often referred to as gay. Homosexual women are usually referred to as lesbians.

There are also people who are attracted to both women and men. These people define their sexuality as bisexual. Bisexual people may have emotional and physical relationships with both men and women during their lives.

Homosexual, bisexual, and heterosexual people all experience emotional attractions to other people. Loving someone else and being loved by someone are wonderful feelings no matter who is feeling them.

These feelings can be confusing. When gay people first begin to realize that they are attracted to people of the same sex, their feelings can be frightening.

Strange Feelings

Daniel remembers the summer he first realized he was gay. "Ben and I had been best friends since the second grade. We did everything together— we lived in the same neighborhood and our families often did things together. We were in the same Scout troop, and we were both on the swim team. We knew everything about each other, and I felt I could tell him anything.

"The summer after eighth grade, Ben met Susan at church camp. When Ben came back from camp, Susan was all he talked about. At first I didn't mind—Susan went to the movies with us, and I thought she was nice. But they were really in love, and when they would hold hands or kiss, I felt uncomfortable—my stomach would get upset, and sometimes I even thought I might throw up. I didn't like Susan taking up so much of Ben's time. That was when I began to realize that I was jealous—I couldn't believe it at first!

"I really felt like my heart was breaking—it was a terrible feeling. I wanted to ask Ben to stop seeing Susan even though I knew that was unfair. I knew if I asked him to break up with her, I'd have

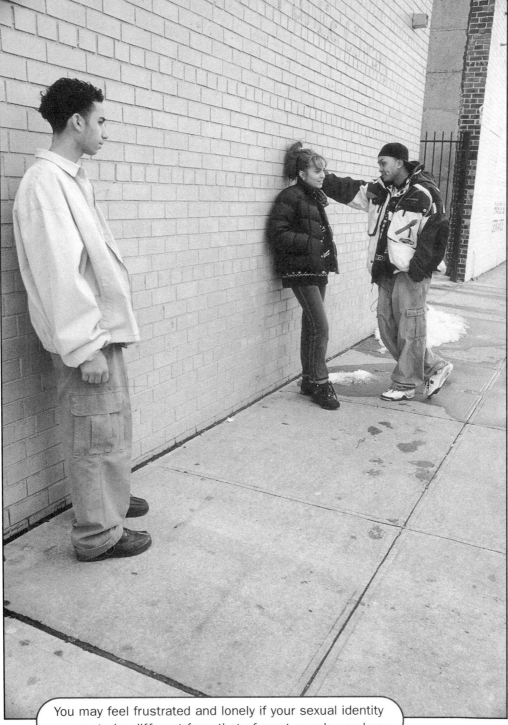

You may feel frustrated and lonely if your sexual identity seems to be different from that of most people you know.

to explain, but I couldn't even explain it to myself. On top of everything else, I was trying to understand why I didn't feel attracted to Susan or to any other girls we knew. I had to admit to myself that I wasn't attracted to girls. I was attracted to Ben."

What Influences Sexual Identity?

Sexual identity is not something that is visible, like the color of your eyes or the length of your hair. It is not possible to know someone's sexual identity by the clothes he or she wears. Straight people look the same as gay and bisexual people do. Gay people come in all shapes, sizes, races, and religions—just like straight people. So what makes their sexual identities different?

In the last few years, scientists have been able to closely study sexual identity. Many of these studies involve genetics. Genetics is the study of genes, which are tiny units of information carried within the cells of your body. Genes carry information that determines the color of your eyes, hair, and skin and all the other qualities of your body. Scientists now believe that genes also carry information that affects your sexual identity. You can't see your genes or choose the ones you want. Your genes are passed on to you from your parents, during the earliest days of your mother's pregnancy.

Knowing that genes affect sexual identity is important because it explains why some people are gay or lesbian and others are not. Some people believe that homosexuals choose to be gay. However, if scientists prove that genes are responsible for sexual identity, then choice is not involved. If you are straight, you probably have never felt that you chose to be attracted to people of the opposite sex. It just happened automatically. Most gay, lesbian, and bisexual people feel the same way. Their sexual identity happened automatically: They did not choose it.

What Do You Want?

It is important to remember that most people want similar things in life. Most people want to live happy lives and pursue careers that satisfy them. Most people want to be able to share their lives in relationships that are loving and caring. This is true no matter what their sexual identity: gay, lesbian, bisexual, or straight.

It is completely normal to have questions or feel confused about your sexual identity. Your sexual identity is not something that is right or wrong. Remember that there are people who can help you sort out your feelings. Your parents, teachers, coaches, and religious leaders are all people who may be able to help you if you are comfortable asking for their help. If you don't feel you can turn to any of those people, there are other places you can go for help. Look at the resource list at the back of this book for phone numbers and addresses of organizations that can help.

Transgendered People

Sexual identity can be a confusing concept. In addition to the sexual identities discussed in this book (gay, straight, lesbian, and bisexual), there is an identity known as *transgender*. Transgender refers to several different groups of people.

Transsexuals are born physically as one sex, but inside they feel that they should be another. Men may feel that they should have been born as women, or women may feel that they should have been born as men. It is now possible to perform surgeries that transform bodies from one sex to another. For someone who is truly transsexual, sex change surgery can greatly improve the quality of his or her life.

Intersexed people are born with a combination of both male and female sex organs. In the past, surgery was performed on intersexed people to make their sex organs just male or just female. Unfortunately, these surgeries were usually performed at a very young age, long before a person was old enough to understand his or her sexual identity. As a result, some intersexed people have found that their bodies were forced into an identity not of their choosing. Doctors are learning to take more time in helping intersexed people to find out what their real sexual identity is.

Crossdressers are people who are comfortable with their gender but who sometimes dress or use mannerisms characteristic of the opposite gender. The word *transvestite* was once used to describe these people, but now crossdresser is the preferred term.

Drag performers (also called *drag queens* and *drag kings*) are performers who dress as members of the opposite sex to entertain audiences. Drag performers are not usually assumed to be transgendered, nor do they always identify themselves as such, since they may be gay or straight and are simply entertainers.

Many transgendered people do not think of themselves as only male or only female; some are comfortable with sexual identities that mix both male and female traits. Many transgendered people are uncomfortable with labeling or naming their sexual identity.

Unfortunately, society has made things very difficult for transgendered people. The movie *Boys Don't Cry* told the true story of Teena Brandon, a transsexual woman who lived her life as a man named Brandon Teena. Sadly, Brandon was raped and murdered when it was discovered that he was really a woman.

We will not discuss transgender issues anywhere else in this book, so please look at the resource list at the back of the book if you think you may be transgendered.

Chapter One

How Do I Know?

If you are reading this book, you may be questioning your own sexual identity. You may feel that you are lesbian or gay without having had any sexual experiences at all. That is OK. Your sexual identity does not require having sex with someone. Remember that sexual identity describes whom you are attracted to with your feelings. Sexual identity is not just physical attraction or a sexual act.

We live in a world that labels people. Even the words gay, lesbian, straight, and bisexual are labels. Though we use labels, sexual identity does not fit into easy categories. Many people who identify themselves as heterosexual adults had emotional or physical relationships with people of the same sex when they were younger. Some homosexual people get married and have children. Each person's life defines his or her sexual identity in a different and very personal way.

Same-Sex Experiences

It is common for young men and young women to have powerful attractions to members of their own sex. This can happen even if the person later grows up to have heterosexual relationships. Sometimes these feelings are a "crush" or strong feelings of attachment to a close friend, favorite teacher, or other special person. Feelings of intense love for someone of the same sex do not automatically mean that someone is gay, though.

Sometimes these are physical, sexual experiences. Not all people have same-sex sexual experiences when they are young, but many people do. Some young girls may kiss a girlfriend while playing dress-up. Young women may press against each other in bed at a slumber party. Some boys may touch each other's bodies in a locker room or while wrestling in the backyard. Sadly, some same-sex experiences may be abusive, such as when a boy is molested by a male relative.

These experiences alone do not mean that the child will grow up to be a lesbian or gay person. It is through both feelings and physical attraction that people begin to define their sexual identities. When your emotional attraction to someone of the same sex is matched by your physical attraction to them, that is an indicator that you might be gay.

Am I Different?

Many lesbian and gay teenagers remember feeling different at a very young age. Some gay teens felt different when they were as young as four and five. If you think you are gay, what are the feelings that led you to believe that? Have you had these feelings for a long time? Do the feelings relate to just one relationship or are they more general feelings?

Lesbian and gay people can be surprised when they begin realizing whom they are attracted to. Since most people in the world are heterosexual, it can be scary to feel like "the only one." While it's normal to be afraid of feeling different, it is also important to understand the reasons you feel that way. Things may not be so frightening if you try to sort things out instead of hiding your feelings from your friends, your family, and even yourself.

Feeling that you are "the only one" can be scary, no matter what the circumstances. For young gay and lesbian people, it's easy to feel that way. The fact is, though, you are not the only one! Statistics indicate that somewhere between 4 and 13 percent of the population identifies itself as gay or lesbian. There may be several million young lesbian and gay people in the United States.

17

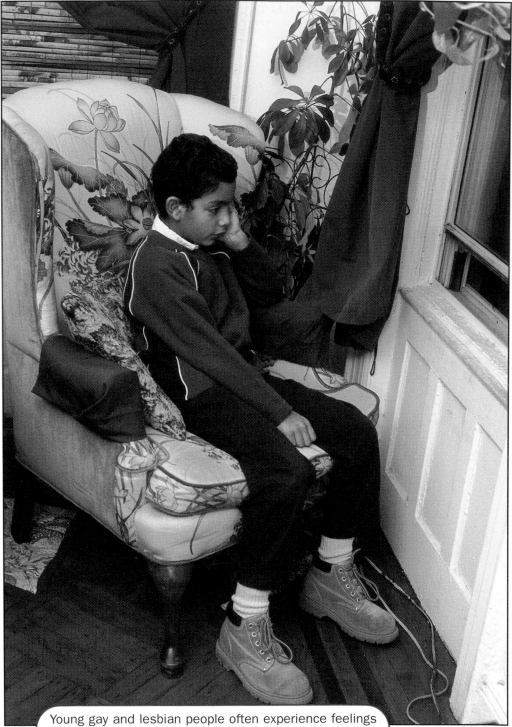

Young gay and lesbian people often experience feelings of isolation, as if they are the only one who is different.

Facing the Truth

Dealing with sexual identity is not easy, especially in a world that does not make it easy for you. Rude jokes are often told about gays or lesbians. President Bill Clinton recently signed a bill that discriminates against gay couples who want to get married. Several people have even been killed because of their sexual identity.

Those are frightening stories, but they are not the only stories about gay and lesbian life. Many lesbians and gays are living with the support of their parents, friends, and family members. Many of them are openly gay at work and are valued by their employers. Even President Clinton has had openly gay advisers! Many lesbian and gay couples are successfully adopting and raising children.

If you discover that you are gay or lesbian or bisexual, try to see that difference as a positive thing. Many people never have the opportunity to think about their lives as deeply as gay and lesbian teens do. It may feel scary, but if you focus on the positive aspects of your personality and your life ahead, you can have a happy and fulfilling life.

Chapter Two

Love and Sex

Love feels wonderful for people of all sexual identities. Being loved by someone we love in return is an important need for everyone. If you are lesbian or gay, it is especially wonderful to connect emotionally with someone who treasures you and understands you. Successful, loving relationships are not easy to find for people of any sexual identity, but they are well worth waiting for.

Sex can be wonderful, too, but it can also be complicated or even dangerous. Sex is a difficult subject for many people to talk about. Religion, fear, and misinformation are some of the reasons people find sex so hard to discuss. As hard as it can be, it is important to talk about sex and the feelings that go along with it. Sex can be wonderful in a loving relationship, but sex itself cannot replace the love you are looking for.

Dating

It is hard to develop healthy loving relationships without getting some practice through dating. Young lesbian and gay people do not have many chances to date other people who share their same-sex attractions. While straight teens are happily asking dates to the prom, gay teens often feel left out. In many places, a lesbian or gay couple can be prevented from attending the prom as a couple!

Fortunately, the dating scene is slowly changing. As more and more teens come out of the closet, fewer people are afraid of lesbian and gay couples. Many colleges—and even some high schools—are forming Gay-Straight Alliances that unite teens of different sexual identities in support of each other. Gay-Straight Alliances sponsor dances and other events that gay couples feel comfortable attending with their partners.

What are the advantages of dating someone? Dating is a process that allows you to get to know somebody. You can share your hopes and dreams with the other person, and they can do the same. Your feelings may grow stronger and deeper, and you might find yourself wanting to be with this person all the time. You may also find that those feelings don't happen. Many good friendships have grown out of relationships that began with dating but did not develop into something else.

When you know someone well, it is easier to make healthy decisions about the relationship. Someone who

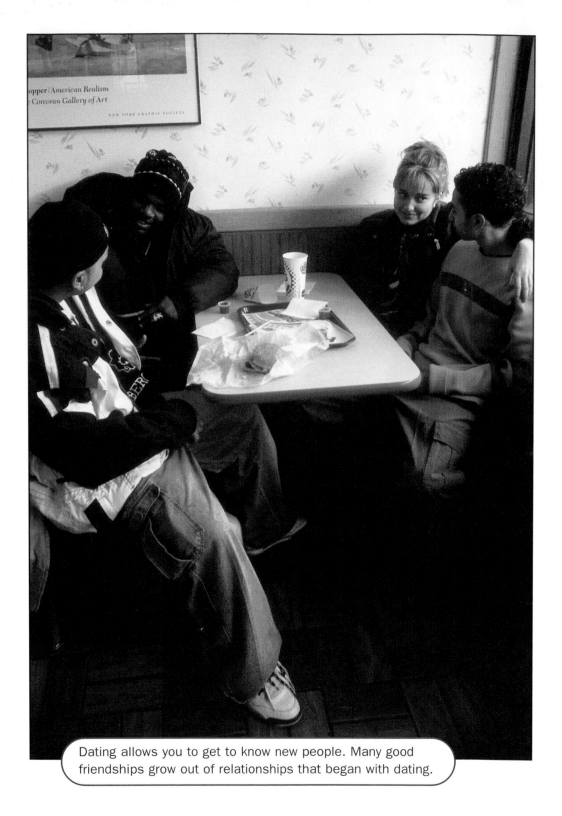

Dating allows you to get to know new people. Many good friendships grow out of relationships that began with dating.

cares enough about you to spend a lot of time with you is probably looking out for your feelings, too. This is especially helpful when a relationship reaches the point where you are considering sex. If you are dating someone who truly cares about you, he or she will not pressure you to have sex. Sex is a big decision. If you do not feel ready for a sexual relationship, then you should not feel embarrassed. If your partner is a caring person, he or she will respect your feelings.

Thinking About Sex

"I was so lucky!" Chyrita explains. "My sister, Deniece, who is straight, first had sex when she was fifteen, and I know it was really hard for her emotionally. The guy who she lost her virginity with didn't really care about her at all. Deniece was really cool when I came out to her, but she begged me to wait to have sex until I was sure it felt right.

"My first long-term relationship with another woman grew out of my relationship with my closest friend, Angela. We met as freshmen during our first year of college. Both of us were very passionate about music, and we spent a lot of time working together at the university radio station. When we weren't actually in class, we spent so much time together that we learned a lot about each other.

"We shared friendly kisses and hugs all the

time, but after several months I knew that I was interested in taking it further. It was nerve-wracking. I didn't know how to talk to her about my sexual feelings, but one night we were having dinner at her place and it was very romantic and we talked enough so that I knew she felt the same way. It just sort of happened naturally that night, and it was very safe and wonderful. Everything I wanted it to be. I was so glad I waited."

Many teens are sexually active in the United States. If you are a gay, lesbian, or bisexual teen who is having sex, it can be really difficult. Not only are you coping with sexual issues, you are also doing so in a society that tries to tell you that your emotions are wrong. That is why it is so important to spend time thinking about what you really want out of love and sex.

In the long run, a strong emotional relationship is far better than a one-night stand. At some point, a loving relationship with another person may begin to include sex as a part of the relationship. If that happens, both partners need to communicate honestly about their desires and concerns. If both partners respect each other's feelings, sex can be a deeply fulfilling part of a relationship. Not all loving relationships have to involve sexual contact, though. There is no right way or wrong way to love someone, as long as the relationship respects the needs and feelings of both people.

Sexually Transmitted Infections (STIs)

Sex can be wonderful, but it can put you at risk for sexually transmitted infections (STIs). These infections are also known as STDs (sexually transmitted diseases) or VD (venereal disease). Nearly three million American teens are diagnosed with a STI every year! STIs are spread from person to person during sexual contact. STIs do not infect people according to their sexual identities. All sexually active people are at risk for STIs.

STIs are caused by bacteria and viruses. Unfortunately, they can be very hard to diagnose because the symptoms are not always obvious. Often the symptoms are very mild or are ignored completely. Your doctor needs to know that you are sexually active in order to look into possible STIs. If you have chosen to be sexually active, you should be sure to let your doctor know so that he or she can help you with the prevention and treatment of an STI. Fortunately, most STIs can now be treated, but you must keep the lines of communication open with your doctor!

A person infected with an STI may not know it. In the case of viral infections, you are infected for life, so it is extremely important to try and prevent infections. Here's a look at some of the most common STIs in the United States.

Chlamydia is the most prevalent STI in the United States. The symptoms are generally very mild—the most common symptom is no symptom at all—and

Herpes, caused by the viruses HSV-1 and HSV-2, can cause sores on the mouth and the genitals. There is no cure, but treatment is available.

many people may have no indication that they have been infected. Chlamydia is caused by bacteria and can be easily treated by a doctor. If chlamydia goes without treatment, though, it can cause sterility in both men and women.

Gonorrhea is another common STI. As with chlamydia, the symptoms in women may be so mild that they are not even noticed. In men, however, the symptoms of gonorrhea are more evident. Symptoms for men include discharge from the penis and severe burning during urination. Gonorrhea is also quite treatable if it is diagnosed early enough. If left untreated, gonorrhea can cause sterility and damage other parts of the body.

Syphilis is also caused by bacteria and can be treated by a doctor. If left untreated, syphilis can cause permanent damage to the heart, brain, skin, bones, or other body organs. The most common symptoms of syphilis are chancre sores. More serious symptoms can include bumpy rashes, peeling skin, large moist spots in the groin, or even large patches of hair loss. In the past, when doctors were not able to treat syphilis with antibiotics, patients eventually became disfigured, blind, or even insane.

Herpes is caused by the viruses HSV-1 and HSV-2. Herpes can cause oozing sores on the mouth and the genital areas, but more important, it can also cause sores that are not even visible! Just touching an infected area can spread herpes, so a condom is not a guarantee of protection. There is no cure, but a doctor can probably treat the sores so that they are not so uncomfortable. Herpes symptoms are periodic, so the sores are not always visible.

Genital warts are caused by the human papilloma virus (HPV). HPV is so common that some experts estimate that one-third of sexually active teens are infected. As with the other STIs mentioned here, you could be infected with HPV for years and spread it to your partners without even knowing it. The warts themselves appear in the genital area, around the penis, anus, or vagina. The flesh-colored warts may be itchy, and they may grow in clusters. The warts can be treated, but the virus cannot. This means that like herpes, HPV is an infection that stays with you for life.

AIDS and HIV

AIDS (acquired immune deficiency syndrome) is an STI you have probably heard a lot about. AIDS is caused by the human immunodeficiency virus, known as HIV. HIV attacks the human immune system. The immune system in your body is what protects you from infection. Your immune system fights viruses (like the common cold) until you get better.

When HIV attacks your immune system, your body is less able to fight off many different diseases. Those diseases together make up the syndrome known as AIDS. There is no cure for HIV or AIDS, and there is no vaccine you can take to prevent an infection. HIV infection *can* be prevented, though, if you take the proper precautions.

HIV can exist in blood, semen, vaginal secretions, and breast milk. HIV can exist in minuscule (extremely small) amounts in tears, sweat, urine, feces, mucus, saliva, and pus, but there are no documented cases of HIV contraction through these fluids. The key to preventing HIV infection is avoiding contact with another person's body fluids that may carry HIV. Many of the possible risks involve sexual contact, but not all of them. Drug users who share needles are at risk because the needles come into direct contact with blood. Mothers who are infected with HIV are at risk of passing the virus on to their babies when they are pregnant or breast-feeding.

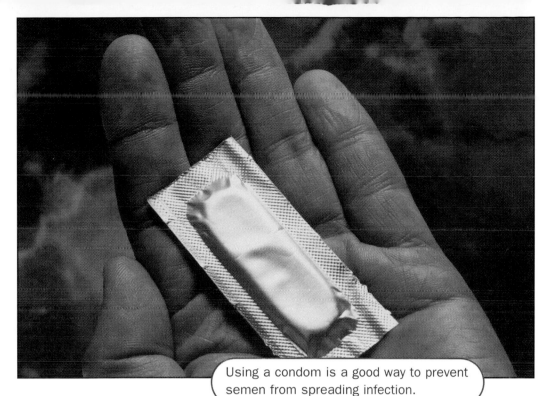

Using a condom is a good way to prevent semen from spreading infection.

Protecting Yourself

In sexual activity, the risk of HIV infection is greatest when dealing with semen, vaginal secretions, and blood. If semen comes in contact with the anus or vagina, there is a risk of infection. If there is even a very small cut or sore on someone's body or in their mouth, there is a risk of infection. It is impossible to know for certain that your partner has no sores just by looking at him or her. Sometimes people can have small cuts or sores inside the anus or vagina where you cannot see them.

HIV can infect you only if it gets inside your body. That means you must prevent your partner's blood, semen, or vaginal secretions from getting inside your body. As with other STIs, a condom is a good way to prevent semen from spreading infection. The condom must not be broken or torn, and it must be used correctly. Condoms are meant for one-time use only. You should never reuse a condom. There are sheets of latex called dams that can be placed across a woman's vagina to prevent contact with her vaginal secretions.

These precautions don't prevent HIV-infected people from enjoying sexual relationships. The precautions prevent the virus from infecting other people. These precautions can also help prevent transmission of other STIs, such as chlamydia, gonorrhea, herpes, syphilis, and genital warts.

Abstinence

The precautions we just talked about are not perfect solutions. Even people who are careful can make a mistake and get an STI. Of course, there are more secure precautions you can take. You can choose to avoid sexual intercourse of any kind. This choice is called abstinence. You can also choose to have no sexual activity at all. This choice is known as chastity.

Abstinence usually means choosing not to engage in specific types of sexual contact. Usually this means no oral, anal, or vaginal intercourse. Some people choose to masturbate together rather than to have sexual intercourse. As long as you are careful not to get your partner's body fluids inside your body, masturbating together can be a very safe sexual activity. Kissing someone you love is wonderful, too, as long as your mouths are free of cuts or sores.

Chastity means not engaging in any kind of sexual behavior with another person. It is possible to have healthy, loving, and fulfilling relationships that do not involve any sexual behavior. How can that be? You can express your love in nonsexual ways. Hugging, dancing, and talking about your feelings are all nonsexual ways of sharing your love with your partner.

Sexual Choices

You are responsible for your own sexual choices. If you choose not to be sexual with someone, that is a healthy, safe choice. Many people wait until they are married or in a long-term relationship before they have any sex at all. There is nothing wrong with being a virgin! There is nothing wrong with making sexual choices, either, if you are truly ready to make them. Choosing to be sexually active means you should also be ready to be a sexually responsible person.

You need to think carefully about the choices that are comfortable for you. Sadly, many people make poor choices in their sexual lives. Sometimes these choices come back to haunt them in the form of STI, emotional problems, or even death. If you have made a sexual choice that is not comfortable for you, stop and think about what you will choose the next time. Remember that you deserve to be loved and treat yourself accordingly.

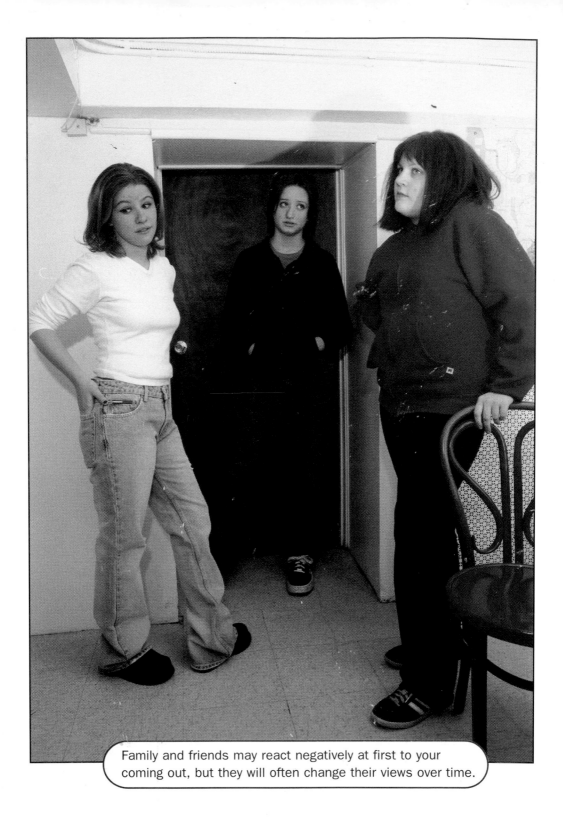

Family and friends may react negatively at first to your coming out, but they will often change their views over time.

Chapter Three | Coming Out

The phrase "coming out of the closet" refers to gay and lesbian people being open and honest about their sexual identity. They "come out" to their families and friends by telling the truth. Most importantly, they are honest with themselves. Coming out is an individual choice. The process is different for each person.

Coming out can be painful. Family and friends do not always react the way you thought they would. For some people, any discussion about homosexuality is very hard. It may be difficult for them to hear the truth. The alternative is to hide the truth or to "stay in the closet." Hiding the truth takes a lot of energy. It requires you to lie about your feelings and desires. Coming out of the closet puts an end to those lies. Coming out is almost always a positive choice in the long run.

Discovering your sexual identity and coming out is also a special opportunity. Many lesbian and gay people feel that they have a chance to explore their feelings more deeply than straight people do. It is an opportunity to learn many things about yourself. The more you know about yourself, the more carefully you can make choices that truly make you happy.

If you are coming out of the closet, there are no rules about how to share your news with family members and friends. Family and friends who react badly at first will often change their views because of their love for you. There are some important things to think about before you come out, though. You need to consider your emotional and physical safety before you begin.

Your Emotional Safety

The circumstances of each person's life are different. You may have been afraid to tell other people that you are lesbian or gay. If that is the case, you need to think about the reasons that you are so afraid. Are you concerned that your parents will stop loving you? Are you afraid that your friends will turn their backs on you?

Family and friends are important pieces of your life. It is important to choose carefully whom you come out to at first. You are sharing something that is deeply personal, so you need to feel safe with the people you are sharing with. For many gays and lesbians, it is easier to tell a friend before breaking the news to family members.

If you are a friend of someone who is gay or lesbian, stand by your friend and help him or her find the courage to be who he or she is. If you are gay or lesbian yourself, reach out for the support you need. Discovering your sexual identity can be a lifelong process. It is not always painful. It is almost always rewarding, though, to find out who you truly are.

Telling a Friend

Trust is an important issue for gays and lesbians still in the closet. As they prepare to tell the truth about themselves, they may be afraid that loved ones will reject them. If you are a friend to someone you think may be lesbian or gay, what can you do? The most important thing is let your friend know that you are a true friend who will be there no matter what. In time, perhaps your friend will feel safe enough to tell you about himself or herself.

Tarren remembers when her best friend, Geoff, came out to her. "It was wintertime. I remember because we were in the car and it was a beautiful, snowy night in February. We were juniors in high school at the time. I had been dating guys for a couple of years by then, but I had never known Geoff to show any interest in girls, although he had a number of close female friends besides me. Geoff and I had never dated, but we had been very close friends and we talked about a lot of things.

"Geoff had been very mysterious earlier that week. I knew there was something on his mind, but whenever I would press him for details he told me he was fine. But on this night, he was kind of nervous and I knew that whatever was bothering him was very important.

"We were headed home after a group dinner with some other friends, and I asked him again what was wrong. He pulled the car over and looked as if he was about to cry. He said he'd been thinking a lot about sharing something with me. And then he turned to me and said, 'Tarren, I'm gay.' I just froze. I wasn't frightened, actually, just sort of overwhelmed by the news. I told him right away that it was OK, that it didn't change anything about our friendship and that I was happy he felt OK about telling me. I asked if he had told anyone else, but he said that I was the first person he'd ever told!

"It was actually very cool that Geoff told me first. I was proud to be a friend that somebody trusted that much because it wasn't just a little thing—this was big news. I told my own parents that night—Geoff knew them very well and I didn't feel it was breaking his confidence to share it with them. My parents were great and told Geoff that they would stand by him if he had any difficulty telling his own parents. I think that set the pattern for Geoff's coming out to other

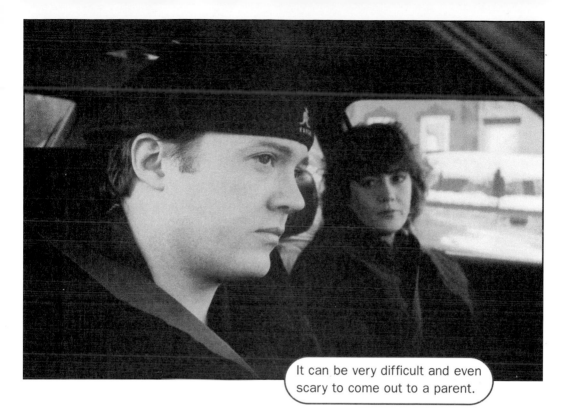

It can be very difficult and even scary to come out to a parent.

people, including everyone in his family. And we are still great friends to this day."

Telling a Parent

It can be very difficult to tell your parents that you are lesbian or gay. Some parents have deep religious beliefs, and they may feel that homosexuality is sinful or wrong. Some parents may feel disappointed or sad that their child's life is not exactly the way they imagined it would be. Sometimes parents are reacting to their own fears for their child's safety and well-being.

When Marga got ready to tell her mother, Luz, that she was a lesbian, she was very frightened. Marga had already come out to her older brother,

37

Paulo, and her sister, Selenia, and they had both accepted her sexual identity. All three children were very close to their mother, but they knew that as a devout Catholic, Luz would have difficulty accepting the news. Still, Marga had begun a relationship with another student, Emily, and she did not want to lie to her mother about it.

One day as Marga visited her mother for lunch, Luz asked a question about Marga's relationship with "her friend." Marga took a deep breath and replied, "Mama, I'm gay."

"I knew it," Luz said, and she sighed. Marga was surprised. Her mother was not throwing a fit, or shouting at her, or even crying.

"Mama, are you angry with me?" Marga asked.

"No, I'm not angry, my love," Luz replied. "I am perhaps disappointed that my dreams for you might not come true. I'm confused that what I've prayed for and what is really happening are not the same thing. But you are my daughter, and I love you very much."

It was not the only time Marga and Luz would talk about their feelings, but it was a good start. Marga felt comfortable introducing Emily to her mother. Luz felt more comfortable with her daughter's life as she got to know Emily better. Marga realized that she had underestimated her mother's love for her.

In many cases, a parent's love for his or her child is more important than his or her feelings about homosexuality. Many parents who react badly at first are able to deal with their feelings without hurting their children. Just as it may take you time to sort out your feelings about coming out, you should remember that the friends and family you tell will need time to sort things out, too.

Your Physical Safety

If you are considering coming out, it is important for you to consider your own physical safety. We live in a world that does not always support people who are honest about their differences. Many African Americans, Hispanics, and other ethnic peoples have suffered discrimination or been subjected to violence because of the color of their skin. For centuries people of different religious beliefs have gone to war. People with physical handicaps have been shunned because their bodies look or work differently. Unfortunately, lesbians and gays have also been subjected to violence.

As frightening as it sounds, many lesbians and gays have been assaulted or even killed simply because they were gay. There are terrible stories of antigay violence occurring all over the United States in recent months and years. Homes and businesses have been bombed, people have been beaten into comas, property has been vandalized, and innocent gay men and women have died. Of course, these things do not happen everywhere. Still, it is a sad fact that you must consider your physical safety before coming out of the closet.

Sadly, one of the places your safety may be most threatened is at school. Most schools in the United States do not have antidiscrimination policies that protect the safety of gay and lesbian teens. There is some good news, though. There are increasing numbers of Gay-Straight Alliances and AIDS awareness clubs as well. If you are comfortable joining (or founding!) a similar club in your own school, that would be a good way to provide yourself with a supportive environment.

Matthew Shepard

Matthew Shepard was a young gay man who lived in Laramie, Wyoming. On October 6, 1998, two local men lured Matthew from a bar. The men drove Matthew to a field outside town, beat him with the butt of a gun, and left him to die, tied to a fence, in near-freezing weather. The two men hid the evidence of their crime and drove back to Laramie, where they assaulted two Hispanic men.

Matthew was discovered the next morning still tied

to the fence, just barely alive. Because of the seriousness of his injuries, Matthew was treated at a hospital
in Fort Collins, Colorado. Sadly, Matthew died in a coma
five days later. He was twenty-one years old.

The two men who murdered Matthew both went to
trial in 1999. Both men could have received the death
penalty for Matthew's murder. Through plea bargains,
both men received sentences of life in prison without
parole. In his remarks following the trial of the second
man, Matthew's father said, "My son has become a
symbol—a symbol for encouraging respect for indi-
viduality; for appreciating that someone is different
[and] for tolerance."

Matthew Shepard's death was reported all over the
world. The story caused many Americans to support
the Hate Crimes Prevention Act, a law that would allow
the FBI to investigate crimes that were committed
because of someone's sexual orientation. Current laws
allow the FBI to investigate a crime that is committed
based on someone's race or religion. As of late 1999,
Congress continued to refuse to pass the Hate Crimes
Prevention Act as long as it included sexual orientation
as one of the categories of hate crimes.

Waiting

If you do not feel safe coming out of the closet to anyone,
you may need to wait until you feel secure. However, you

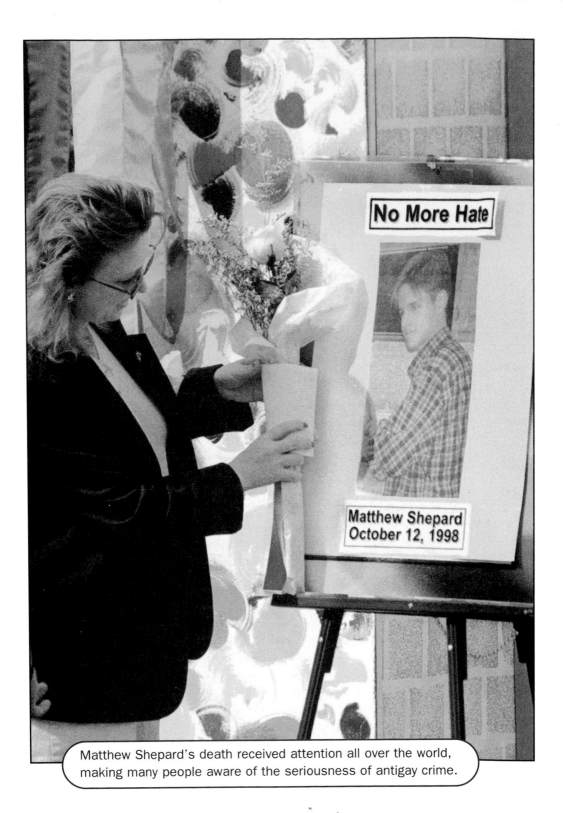

Matthew Shepard's death received attention all over the world, making many people aware of the seriousness of antigay crime.

can still reach out for help. You can try reaching out to a teacher, counselor, or even a church leader if any of these options feel safe to you.

Look at the resource list at the end of the book. When you call one of the organizations listed, it should be able to direct you to resources in your local area.

Chapter Four

Someone to Look Up To

If you are just figuring out your own sexual identity, it is easy to feel like "the only one." Many people have struggled with their sexual identities. Many other people have supported lesbian and gay friends or family members. Here are stories about just a few of those people.

Wilson Cruz

Wilson Cruz is a young actor who has been openly gay since the beginning of his career. He plays Victor on the TV series *Party of Five* and has performed on Broadway in the musical *Rent*. In 1994, Wilson became well known for playing a gay character on the TV show *My So-Called Life*. The character he played, Rickie

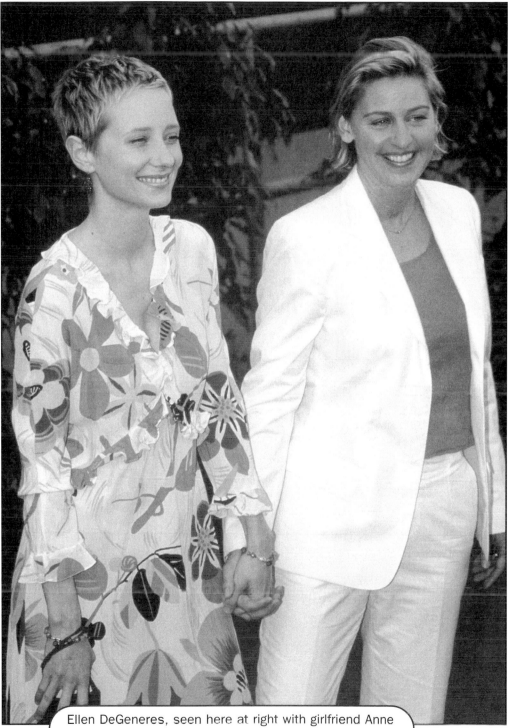

Ellen DeGeneres, seen here at right with girlfriend Anne Heche, was the first openly gay star of her own TV show.

Vasquez, was a gay high school student struggling to cope. It was a role that hit close to home because Wilson's Puerto Rican family did not deal well with his coming out of the closet. His father kicked him out of the house when he told them he was gay.

"I think back to the times I tried to slit my wrists, times I tried to just end it because I didn't know anyone else was going through it," Wilson told *Advocate* magazine in 1994. "I would turn on the TV and think, please give me a sign that I fit in somewhere, that I'm not alone out here. I hope I can help kids see that they're not the only ones in the world." Wilson is an amazing young man with a bright future ahead of him. He will soon appear on the big screen with Angela Bassett and Lou Diamond Phillips in the movie *Supernova*.

Ellen and Betty DeGeneres

Ellen DeGeneres is a comedian and actress who came out of the closet on her own TV show, *Ellen*. The character Ellen played on the show had never had a major romantic interest. After several seasons, DeGeneres decided she would like her sitcom to mirror her personal life. In the mid-1990s, Ellen decided to come out of the closet as a lesbian in both her public and her private life.

At the time, there had not been many major gay or lesbian characters on television. While gays often appeared as supporting characters in shows like

Friends or *My So-Called Life,* there had never been a gay or lesbian leading character on television. The producers of Ellen's show at ABC were reluctant to let her pursue the lesbian storyline. However, Ellen used her power as the star of the show to create a storyline in which her character, Ellen Morgan, discovered her true sexual identity. Ellen also began doing interviews in which she told the truth about her own life and her loving relationship with the actress Anne Heche.

Ellen's mother, Betty DeGeneres, was supportive of Ellen's choice to come out publicly. Ellen had come out to her mother many years earlier, and they had worked through many of their difficult feelings. Betty even made a TV appearance on the episode of *Ellen* where her daughter's character first says, "I'm gay." Recently, Betty wrote the book *Love, Ellen: A Mother-Daughter Journey.* Betty has appeared publicly to support her daughter and encourage other people to come out to their families. "I hope that one day it will not seem so exceptional that a mother would show equal concern for her gay and straight children," Betty has said. "I see it as a simple matter of common sense, common decency, and love."

Audre Lorde

Audre Lorde described herself as a "black lesbian, mother, warrior, poet." She earned degrees at both Hunter

College and Columbia University and was a great teacher and writer. Audre was a social activist who dedicated herself to a number of causes: civil rights, celebration of African-American culture, and gay and lesbian rights, to name just a few. "When I dare to be powerful—to use my strength in the service of my vision, then it becomes less and less important whether I am afraid," Audre wrote. She died of breast cancer in 1992 at the age of fifty-eight.

Rudy Galindo

"Stick to your dreams," Rudy Galindo said when asked to offer advice to fellow Mexican Americans. "I did, and look at me." The world has been looking at Rudy ever since he won the men's title in the National Figure Skating Championship in early 1996. It was not an easy road to success for this openly gay skater. In the early 1990s, Kristi Yamaguchi broke away from her successful skating partnership with Rudy to pursue her own solo career. His father died of a heart attack in 1993, and AIDS took the lives of two of his skating coaches and one of his brothers.

Still, Rudy continued to pursue the sport he loves and finally won the national title at the age of twenty-six. In his autobiography, *Icebreaker,* Rudy writes honestly about his sexual identity, as well as his struggles with drugs and poverty. His life is truly inspiring for anyone who wants to focus on following his or her dreams.

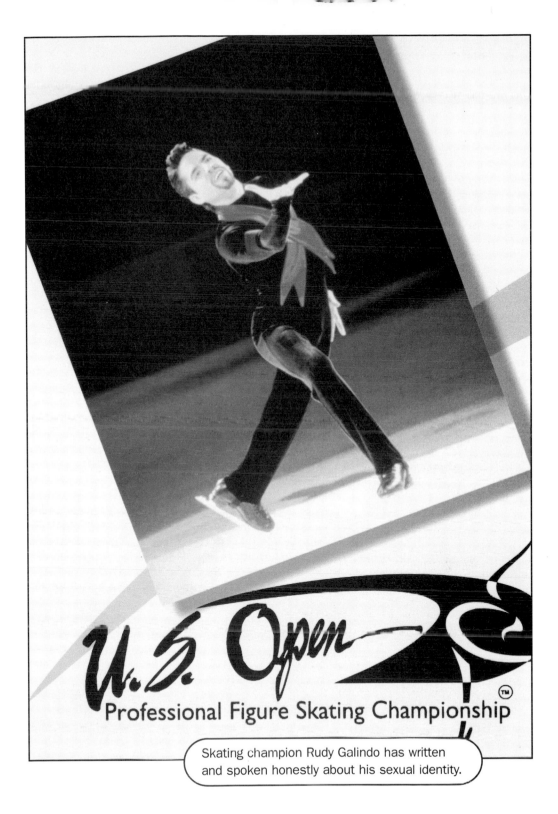

U.S. Open
Professional Figure Skating Championship ™

Skating champion Rudy Galindo has written and spoken honestly about his sexual identity.

The Galluccio Family

Jon and Michael Galluccio fell in love as college students in the early 1980s. They knew immediately that they were life partners. Though their parents were not accepting of them when they came out of the closet, they both became successful professionals in New York City. Eventually they moved to a small suburb in New Jersey to begin raising a family. Both Jon and Michael applied to the state of New Jersey to become foster and adoptive parents.

Their first child, Adam, was placed with them in late 1995. Adam was two months old and had a number of serious health problems, including HIV-infection and a damaged heart. Adam was nursed back to health under their care. However, when Jon and Michael applied to adopt Adam, they were told that would be impossible. Under the state's laws, Jon and Michael were considered an unmarried couple and therefore not allowed to adopt. (The same rule would have applied if they were an unmarried man and woman.)

Jon and Michael knew that unless they were allowed to adopt Adam, he could be removed from their home at any time. The state of New Jersey continued to consider Jon and Michael acceptable foster parents. The state placed another young boy, Andrew, in their care. Jon and Michael filed a lawsuit against the state of New Jersey and won the right for unmarried couples—

including gay and lesbian couples—to be considered as adoptive parents on the same grounds as married heterosexual couples. Though Andrew was eventually returned to his natural grandparents, Jon and Michael adopted Adam in 1997. Since then the Galluccios have adopted two daughters, Madison and Rosa.

Chapter Five

The Life Ahead of You

"T*he worst part was that I was really depressed, and I didn't know who to talk to. If it had been about anything else, I would have talked to my mom about it, but I couldn't do that. My parents knew something was wrong, but I didn't know what to say to them. I stopped going out, and I couldn't really remember feeling happy. That was when my mom asked me if I wanted to talk to a therapist."*

Getting Help

Despite the challenges of being lesbian, gay, or bisexual, there are many places you can turn for help.

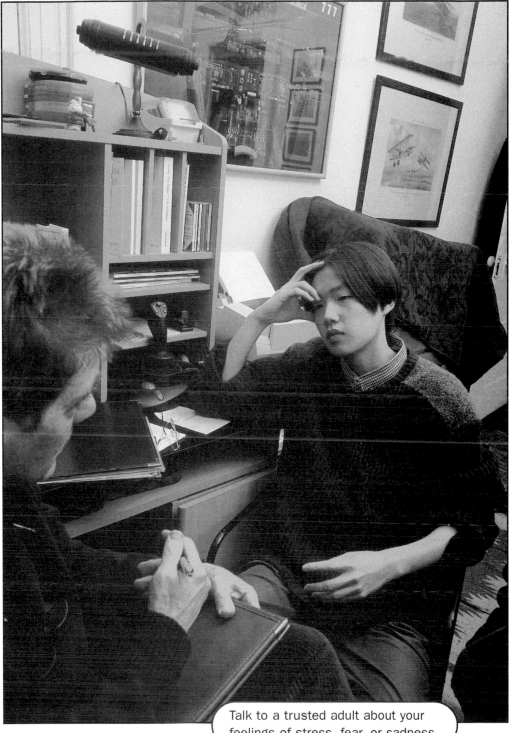

Talk to a trusted adult about your feelings of stress, fear, or sadness.

You may find yourself dealing with feelings of stress, fear, sadness, or anger. If that is the case, you should try to speak with someone about your feelings. Perhaps you can talk with a friend or relative. If not, you should try to find a counselor, clergyperson, or support group to talk to. You can also use the resource list at the back of this book. Many organizations have toll-free numbers or Web sites you can use to get more information or support in your area.

What's Next?

Coming out is not a one-time event. For many people, sexual identity is an issue that they deal with throughout their lives. The good news is that things are slowly changing for the better. More and more positive images of gay, lesbian, and bisexual people can be seen in the world at large. In television, movies, advertising, and magazines, people of all sexual identities are more visible than ever before. These images are becoming truer to life, with gay characters facing the same life challenges as their straight counterparts.

Surround yourself with people who support you and the things you believe. If you are lucky, these people are your family members who love you deeply. If you cannot find the support you need from your family, then reach out to friends. Somewhere along the way you will find the support and encouragement you need.

Having the courage to be yourself will help you lead a fulfilling life.

Gay, lesbian, and bisexual people are all races, religions, and sexes. They can be anything they want to be. They can be lawyers, doctors, teachers, parents, dancers, writers, or a thousand other things. Gay, lesbian, and bisexual people can be just as happy and fulfilled as their straight friends and family. With the courage to come out and be who they truly are, they will all lead fulfilling lives.

Glossary

anal intercourse Sexual interaction in which the penis enters the anus.

bisexual Someone who is attracted to both men and women.

chlamydia A bacteria that can infect mucus membranes in the penis, vagina, cervix, anus, urethra, or eye.

gay A common word meaning homosexual, or someone who is attracted to people of the same sex.

genital warts Warts caused by the human papilloma virus (HPV) that cause flesh-colored cauliflower bumps on the penis, vulva, anus, mouth, or vagina.

gonorrhea A sexually transmitted infection that can cause sterility, arthritis, heart problems, and blindness in newborns.

herpes An infection that can be sexually transmitted and causes a recurring rash with clusters of sores on the vagina, cervix, penis, mouth, anus, buttocks, or elsewhere on the body.

lesbians Women who are attracted to other women; female homosexuals.

masturbation Touching one's own sex organs for pleasure.

oral intercourse Sexual interaction in which the penis enters the mouth.

syphilis A sexually transmitted infection that can lead to disfigurement, skeletal damage, neurological illness, or death.

transgender Term used to describe people who do not think of themselves as only male or only female or who are uncomfortable with labeling or naming their sexual identity.

transvestite Someone who dresses in clothing characteristic of the opposite sex.

vaginal intercourse Sexual interaction in which the penis enters the vagina.

vaginal secretions Fluids produced inside the vagina.

Where to Go for Help

In the United States

Human Rights Campaign
1101 14th Street NW, Suite 200
Washington, DC 20005
(202) 628-4160
Web site: http://www.hrc.org

National AIDS Hotline
(800) 342-AIDS

National Coming Out Project
(800) 866-6263

National Gay and Lesbian Task Force
2320 17th Street NW
Washington, DC 20009

(202) 332-6483
Web site: http://www.ngltf.org

National Latino/a Lesbian and Gay Organization
1612 K Street NW, Suite 500
Washington, DC 20006
(202) 466-8240
Web site: http://www.llego.org

Parents and Friends of Lesbians and Gays (PFLAG)
1101 14th Street NW, Suite 1030
Washington, DC 20005
(202) 638-4200
Web site: http://www.pflag.org

In Canada

Canadian Gay, Lesbian, and Bisexual Resource Directory
Web site: http://www.gaycanada.com

Canadian Queer Resources Directory
Web site: http://www.qrd.org/world/americas/canada

Equality for Gays and Lesbians Everywhere (EGALE)
306-177 Nepean Street
Ottowa, ON K2P OB4
(613) 230-1043
Web site: http://www.egale.ca

Transgender Resources

American Education Gender Information Service
(AEGIS)
P.O. Box 33724
Decatur, GA 30033-0724
e-mail: aegis@mindspring.com
Web site: http://www.gender.org/aegis

International Foundation for Gender Education
(IFGE)
P.O. Box 540229
Waltham, MA 02454-0229
(781) 899-2212

Web Sites

GenderPAC
http://www.gpac.org

!OutProud! The National Coalition for Gay, Lesbian,
and Bisexual Youth
http://www.outproud.org

Planned Parenthood
http://www.teenwire.com

Queer Resources Directory
http://www.qrd.org

For Further Reading

Bass, Ellen, and Kate Kaufman. *Free Your Mind: The Book for Gay, Lesbian, and Bisexual Youth—and Their Allies*. New York: HarperCollins, 1996.

DeGeneres, Betty. *Love, Ellen: A Mother-Daughter Journey*. New York: Rob Weisbach Books, 1999.

Due, Linnea. *Joining the Tribe: Growing Up Gay and Lesbian in the 90s*. New York: Anchor Books, 1995.

Galindo, Rudy. *Icebreaker: The Autobiography of Rudy Galindo*. New York: Pocket Books, 1997.

Gibson, Scott, ed. *Blood and Tears: Poems for Matthew Shepard*. New York: Painted Leaf Press, 1999.

Lorde, Audre. *A Burst of Light: Essays*. Ithaca, NY: Firebrand Books, 1998.

Mastoon, Adam. *The Shared Heart: Portraits and Stories Celebrating Lesbian, Gay, and Bisexual Young People*. New York: William Morrow, 1997.

Stewart, Gail. *Gay and Lesbian Youth*. San Diego, CA: Lucent Books, 1997.

Index

A

abstinence, 30–31
adoption, 19, 50–51
AIDS/HIV, 28, 29–30, 48, 50
AIDS awareness clubs, 40
anger, feelings of, 54
antidiscrimination policies,
    40
antigay violence, 39–40
attraction
    emotional, 7, 8, 16–17
    physical/sexual, 7, 8, 15,
        16–17

B

bisexuality, definition of, 8
Boys Don't Cry, 14
Brandon, Teena, 14

C

chastity, 30, 31
chlamydia, 25–26, 30

Clinton, Bill, 19
coming out, 32–34, 41–43,
    54
    emotional safety, 34–35
    physical safety, 39–40
    to a friend, 35–37
    to a parent, 37–39
communication, 24, 25
condoms, 27, 29–30
confusion, 9, 12
counselors, 43, 54
crossdressers, 13–14
Cruz, Wilson, 44–46

D

dating, 7, 21–23
DeGeneres, Ellen and Betty,
    46–47
drag performers, 14

E

Ellen, 46–47

Index

F
fear of being different, 17
fear of rejection, 34, 35

G
Galindo, Rudy, 48
Galluccio, Jon and Michael, 50–51
Gay-Straight Alliances, 21, 40
genetics, 11–12
genital warts/human papilloma virus (HPV), 27, 30
gonorrhea, 26, 30

H
Hate Crimes Prevention Act, 41
Heche, Anne, 47
herpes, 27, 30
homosexuality, definition of, 8

I
identity, 6–7
intersexed people, 13

K
kissing, 7, 16, 30–31

L
Lorde, Audre, 47–48
love, 7, 8, 16, 20, 24, 31, 34, 39

M
masturbation, 30

P
parents, 12, 19, 34, 37–39

R
religion/religious beliefs, 20, 37, 39
religious leaders/clergy-person, 12, 43, 54

S
same-sex experiences, 16–17
sex, 7, 15, 20, 23, 24, 29–31
  dangers of, 25–28
sex change surgery, 13
sexual identity, definition of, 7–8
sexual identity, influences on, 11–12
sexually transmitted infections (STIs), 25–28, 29–30, 31
Shepard, Matthew, 40–41
stress, feelings of, 54
support groups, 54
syphilis, 27, 30

T
teachers, 12, 43
transgendered people, 13–14
transsexuals, 13
transvestites, 14

V
venereal disease (VD), 25
virginity, 23, 31

About the Author

Jeff Donaldson-Forbes is a playwright and author living on the east coast. He has volunteered with Gay Men's Health Crisis in New York City and worked with AIDS-related community services in upstate New York.

Photo Credits

Cover by Ira Fox; p. 26 © Custom Medical Stock Photo; p. 29 © Index Stock; p. 41 © Reuters/Gary Caskey/ Archive Photos; pp. 44, 48 © The Everett Collection; all other photos by Bob Van Lindt.